Healthy Eating to Gain Muscles & Healthy Weight

Healthy Eating to Gain Muscles

and

Healthy Weight

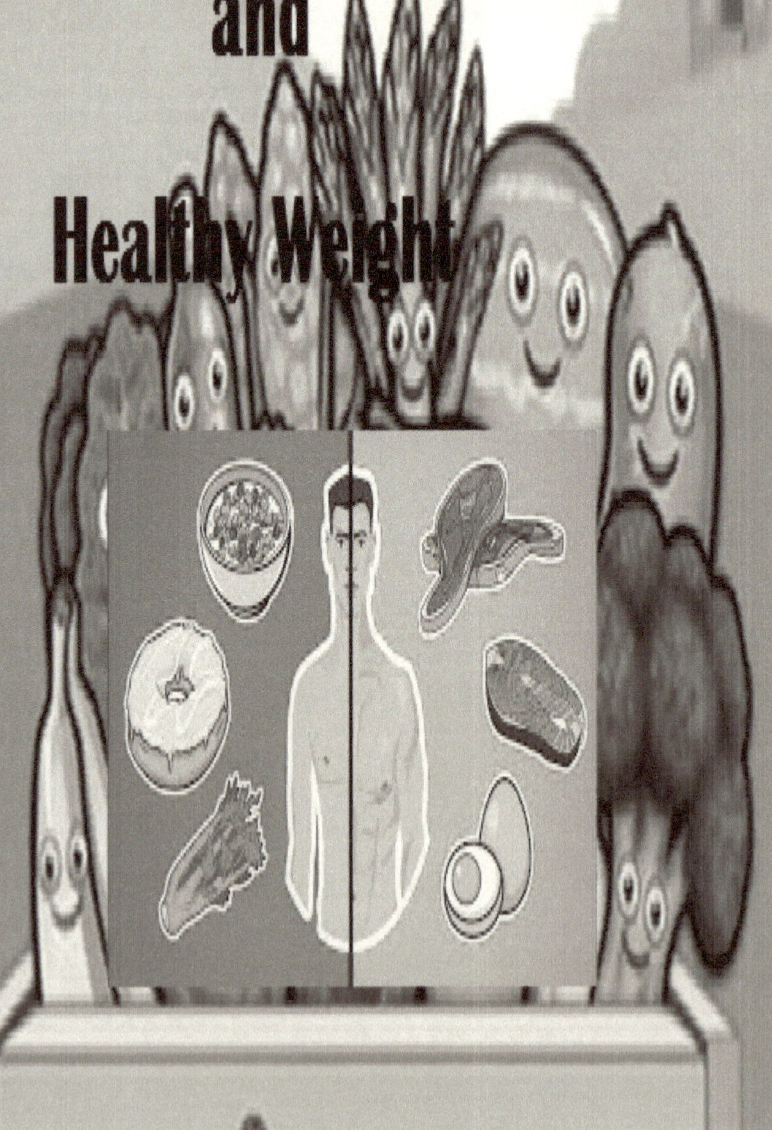

<u>Table of Contents</u>

Introduction

Healthy eating starts by being conscious of our behavior and attitude towards the food that we are about to eat. This is through the philosophy of mindful eating, which most people do not give importance. Usually we sit down and start eating, but not keen about how the food was grown, harvested and transported to the market and to our dinner plate.

This book "Healthy Eating to Gain Muscles & Healthy Weight" will give you tips on how to begin the art of mindful eating, its basics and as you develop it, you will be amazed at how it can change your outlook towards appreciating the food, and how it can make you healthy.

This book also guides you on the different diet programs and food choices that can help increase your muscle mass and lose weight. It is up to you to decide which of the diet programs are suited to your lifestyle, dietary requirements and food preferences.

There is no perfect diet program, but one thing for sure is that each has the ability to lose weight and lower the risks of heart disease, diabetes, cancer, alleviates inflammation and improves insulin sensitivity.

All these aspects are covered in this eBook based on some studies that could prove their effectiveness in the battle against obesity, which is a growing health problem affecting both adults and children. Each diet plan emphasizes the importance of eating fruits, vegetables, whole grains, nuts, and seeds.

This book provides answers to your questions on how to get started with a diet plan to lose weight and eat the right foods that help build muscle.

Let's get started!

Chapter 1: Healthy Eating Plan for Beginners

Most people are gaining weight despite their effort to curb their extra pounds as they do not know where to start. Staying healthy begins with a healthy eating plan. This is according to a statement issued by the Dietary Guidelines for Americans 2015-2020. The healthy eating plan involves a healthy balance of the following:

- Focus on vegetables, fruits, whole grains, seeds, and fat-free or reduced-fat milk products, preferably plant-based milk.
- Avoid red meats; instead eat lean meats, fish, poultry, eggs, nuts, and beans as your source of protein.
- Choose foods that are low in trans fats, cholesterol and saturated fats.
- Stay away from high sodium and sugary foods.
- Follow your daily calorie needs.

Having a healthy eating plan can help a lot in managing your desired weight based on your age and height. This plan includes a variety of whole-food, plant-based foods that you often dislike as you've been eating unhealthy and processed foods for the past decades. Since you noticed that you gained a lot of weight, you decided to focus on healthy eating.

Here are some foods to consider for your weekly menu plan.

1. Rainbow-colored foods

Adding a variety of multi-colored vegetables to your dinner plate is your first step towards healthy eating. Among the foods that you can choose are dark, leafy green veggies, tomatoes, oranges, onions, carrots, bell peppers, arugula, broccoli, cauliflower, grapes, and fresh herbs like dill, rosemary, and thyme for your salad greens. Omelets, soups and stews taste so good if you add some vegetables and fresh herbs, which are loaded with antioxidants, fiber, minerals and vitamins.

2. Try fresh, canned or frozen fruits

Fruits offer a variety of nutrients and water contents to keep you hydrated while working out. If you love exotic fruits and they are not available in your place, try looking for canned or frozen fruits in grocery shelves, such as pineapple, durian, papayas, mangosteen, mangoes, and kiwis. Make sure to read the label and look for canned varieties packed in their own juice or water and avoid canned fruits that have added syrups and sugars, which can defeat your purpose of losing weight.

3. Try a different way to prepare the veggies

If you dislike vegetables, you can prepare them in a variety of ways to suit your impeccable taste buds. Aside from salad greens, try grilling or steaming the vegetables and add some herbs and spices to enhance their taste and dip the veggies in sauce or dips. Pan-frying, roasting, baking or stir-frying are other cooking methods that you can think of to make your vegetable dish pleasing to your taste buds. When using canned veggies, look for products that have no added sugars, cream sauces, salt, or butter if you want to stay fit.

4. Add calcium-rich foods

Calcium rich foods are important to keep your bones healthy while trying to reduce weight through strength training or bodyweight exercises. When you are exercising, injury can be avoided if your body is sufficient in calcium. Look for low-fat or reduced-fat or fat-free milk and yogurt without added sugars.

5. Try different cooking methods

Frying or sautéing are not always recommended, why not use another cooking method in preparing your fish, chicken or turkey. Try roasting, grilling, searing or baking them for variation. If you are really bent on reducing your weight, you can even replace the meat with beans as your source of protein and fats. There are a variety of beans and legumes that you can prepare for your protein and healthy fat needs.

Having a healthy eating plan does not deprive you of your favorite comfort foods as healthy eating is not about deprivation, but it emphasizes on balanced diet. You can still eat high calorie, fatty and sugary foods, but not always. Balance out your comfort food with healthy and nutritious foods alongside with your daily physical activity.

If you've been eating your comfort food daily, cut back to once per week or even once per month if you want to cut your calorie intake. Eat them in smaller portions, say half or ¼ of a bar, instead the entire bar. When cooking your pasta dish, use low calorie ingredients. Try using non-fat milk instead of whole milk or use light cream cheese and less butter. Cutting back on calories is one step ahead in maintaining a healthy weight while still enjoying your comfort food.

Chapter 2: Mindful Eating for Weight Loss

Mindful eating is not only centered on the kind of food that you are eating, but on your behavior towards eating. By paying attention to your eating moment, it can help improve your health by managing your diet, food cravings, and losing weight.

What is Mindful Eating?

Mindful eating is a philosophy that focuses on the in-the-moment awareness of the food and drinks that you take. While eating, you don't have to judge how the food or drinks make you feel and the body signals regarding satiation, taste, and satisfaction. Under this philosophy, you acknowledge and learn to accept the bodily sensations, feelings, and thoughts that you observe which also include how you bought, prepare, serve, and consume the food. Mindful eating includes the following:

- Letting yourself aware of the nurturing and positive opportunities that come to you through the right selection of food and how it is prepared by following your inner wisdom.
- When choosing what to eat, use your senses to find food that brings nourishment and satisfaction to your body.
- You acknowledge your bodily responses without judging how the food or drink reacts to your body.
- You learn to identify between satiety and physical hunger cues as your guide in making decisions on how to start and finish eating.

Most people have no time for food preparation because of their fast-paced life and quick meals are the only thing they can prepare using grocery-bought ingredients that are heavily processed. During mealtime, we often get distracted with our hectic schedule, so we eat mindlessly, slurping the food as if it is our last, then answering calls and realizing later that we have eaten much regardless if we are hungry or not.

Sometimes when we feel dizzy while working at our desk, we keep our mouth busy with potato chips or tortillas even if we are not really hungry. Our busy lives make us gain weight that leads to obesity and develop later to a serious medical condition like diabetes and cardiovascular disease. Some people use food as their outlet to satisfy their emotional needs and as a coping mechanism when they are beset with problems or to beat boredom.

Mindful eating on the other hand, though not perfect, it can help reduce weight as you eat slowly, which is recommended by health experts to make your stomach fully satisfied and delay hunger as the food is masticated in the mouth for a several seconds. Eating-on-the go is discouraged in mindful eating as you are taught to eat the right food and not allowing yourself to eat everything that your heart desires, but in a slow pace and focused all your senses.

Mindful eating does not require you to follow strict rules on your calorie intake or what type of food you are going to eat and avoid, but on observing your manner of eating, how the food is presented when you shop, prepare, serve and consume. As you are accustomed to this philosophy, your body is attuned to it, and you will be able to avoid careless eating, overeating, and binge eating, which ultimately can help shift to a dietary habit that can improve your mental and physical health.

What are the Benefits of Mindful Eating?

Mindful eating is an effective method of combating food-related behaviors, eating disorders and habits that make a person gain weight. Adapting mindfulness in eating is similar to mindfulness in the Buddhist philosophy, where you are taught to discipline your mind and body. Through mindful eating you will discover the root cause of your eating disorders, food cravings and learn how to correct them using your feelings, physical cues and experiences.

Here are the benefits you get from mindful eating:

- You will be able to learn the art of slow eating for proper digestion.
- You know if you are really hungry by listening to physical hunger cues.
- You learn how to eat until full, and not eating carelessly.
- You are able to identify between true hunger and non-hunger triggers for eating.
- You are able to cope with guilt, anxiety and behavioral problems about food.
- You are able to engage your senses on how to detect the flavors, texture, tastes and color of the food.
- You eat right to stay healthy and reduce weight.

- You learn how to appreciate the food and not judging how it reacts to your body as well as avoid overeating.
- You are able to determine how the food can affect your feelings and appearance.
- You learn how to slow down and take a break from your busy day.
- You make healthier choices of your food after focusing on how you feel after eating the food.
- You feel connected to the source of your food and how it was brought to the market.

Tips on How to Practice Mindful Eating

Mindful eating can be learned by participating in an activity using your total awareness by paying attention to what you are doing. Say for example, when you eat, focus on the food, and avoid any distractions by putting away your gadgets, books or iPhone. Set a schedule for TV watching, chatting, and reading instead of doing it all together while dining. When your mind roams somewhere else, go back to your food and rekindle the moment how it was bought, prepared and served.

Tips to Get Started with Mindful Eating:

1. Take mindfulness slowly, by doing it briefly for your first try. A five-minute period is just enough on your first meal of the day and then increase the time in your next meal. Take note that when you buy the food, or browsing the recipe online, you can of course start the first step of mindful eating. When checking on the menu or recipe, make an assessment of each item before adding to your cart or list.

2. Next, take a few deep breaths while thinking about the nutrients you get from each food item. If you are about to pick the item from the grocery shelves, breathe in and then exhale and imagine how you become healthier with the kind of food that you are going to shop. With

this kind of attitude, you return those items that are not good for your health, and swap them with nutritious food instead.

3. Use all your senses while shopping, preparing the food, serving and eating. Observe how the food, say vegetable look like and smell while chopping it. How they sound while stirring them in hot oil and how it taste after putting the seasonings.

4. Observe yourself and the food you are about to partake of. Pay attention to how you are seated, make sure to sit properly and relaxed, and feel your surroundings and remove all the distractions while you are in the process of eating and enjoy the experience.

5. Ask yourself if you are hungry when you come to the table. If not, don't start eating. The purpose of eating is you are really hungry in the true sense of the word, and not merely addressing to your hunger pangs and cravings for the sake of eating.

6. Appreciate the food in front of you and the people who will be sharing the meal. Take a close look at the shapes, textures, aroma, and colors of the dishes. Feel your reaction to the food presentation. What is in the food that you like most?

7. Taste the food by taking a bite. Observe how your tongue feels the taste and the texture. Identify what's in the dish, its ingredients, and flavors. After biting, start chewing the food and differentiate the taste and texture.

8. Concentrate on your experience every time you eat the food. Are you gratified and happy with what you are eating? Eat your food slowly with presence of mind and don't rush to catch up your other commitments of the day.

9. After each bite, put your spoon and fork down and contemplate your experience if you are hungry or satiated before taking another bite. Always listen to your stomach and what you put into your plate. Know where to stop eating.

10. Be thankful and contemplate on the source of the food, the creator, the plants and animals used in the production of food and the farm workers and those involved in transporting the food to the market and to your plate. Minding the food sources can help you make wise and sustainable decisions that is not only for your good health, but for the environment as well.

11. Lastly, keep eating slowly while you can now start chatting with your family or friends at the table, while paying attention if you are full and satisfied. Whether you are with your dining companions or eating alone, never forget to stay focused on your present experience while finishing your meal.

Mindful eating is a discipline similar to physical exercise where every step matters most. The more effective you are in doing this mental and emotional training, the better you become as a person, and most of all in maintaining a healthy body as you learn to appreciate and consume the food when you are hungry and not to satisfy your cravings while taking control of your dietary habits.

Chapter 3: Types of Diet Programs for Weight Loss

Your friends are boasting their diet programs, and you want to follow suit, but you are a bit confused which diet plan is best for you. Changing your diet could be tricky knowing that there are countless of diet plans available today as you are not sure which of them works best for your body and age. Some diets differ in their regimen and methodology, and before you start dieting, you have to familiarize with a number of diet plans.

Here are some diet programs that might suit to your lifestyle and needs.

1. Plant-Based Diets

Consuming plant-based foods can reduce weight without exerting much effort. Followers of vegan and vegetarianism claim they are able to maintain their weight by eating fruits and vegetables and avoidance of animal products like meat and dairy not only for health but for environmental and ethical reasons.

There are many versions of plant-based diets, such as whole-food, plant-based (WFPB) diet, which discourage heavily manufactured food and animal products in the diet. An example is the flexitarian diet, which allows eating meat and its byproducts in moderation along with fruits and vegetables. If you follow this diet, you can still eat meat in moderation and focus on eating fruits, veggies, legumes, and whole grains.

There are numerous studies that show the benefits of a plant-based diet. A review of twelve studies involving 1,151 participants revealed that those who relied on a plant-based diet were able to lose about 4.4 pounds than those who eat animal products. Followers of a vegan diet were able to reduce an average of 5.5 pounds than those who did not eat a plant-based diet. The reason is pretty obvious as plant-based diets are rich in fiber that can make your stomach feel full and low in calorie fat. A plant-based diet can reduce the risk of heart disease, diabetes and cancers.

2. Low-carb diets

There are many variations of low-carb diets, such as Ketogenic diet, high-fat (LCHF), low-carb, and Atkins diet. In general, these diet plans are centered on reducing carbohydrates in the diet and focus on fat and protein to reduce weight, but they have some characteristics that could differentiate each other. For example, Keto or Ketogenic diet restricts carbohydrates in the diet to ten percent or below of your total calories compared to other versions of low carb diet which restricts 30 or less percent of the total calories.

Proponents of low-carb diets claim that adding more protein in the diet can curb the appetite, increase metabolism and save your muscle mass. If you choose a Ketogenic diet, your body starts using fatty acids instead of carbohydrates for fuel by turning them into ketones through the process of ketosis. Numerous studies show that low-carb diets can help in weight reduction and more effective than traditional low fat diets.

In fact, a review of about 53 studies involving 68,128 participants showed that people who submit to low carb diets lost more weight than those who resorted to low-fat diets. Low-carb diets are found to be more effective in burning your belly fat and it can reduce the risk factors for cardiovascular diseases, high blood cholesterol, and blood sugar level.

3. Intermittent Fasting

Intermittent fasting is one of the most popular diets in today's generation because it is easy to implement. It uses the cycles between the periods of eating and fasting, which means you can fast for 16 hours, including your sleeping period and then enjoy your food in the remaining eight hours. This is under the 16/8 method. If you choose the 5:2 fasting method, you are required to limit your calorie intake from 500 to 600 only twice each week.

The philosophy behind intermittent fasting is that you are restricted to eating only within a certain time window as a way to reduce calorie intake. If done regularly, you are able to reduce your weight provided you don't each much during your eating periods.

Based on some studies, intermittent fasting can reduce about 3 to 8 percent of weight in a period from 3 to 24 weeks, which is far better than other diet plans. It targets your waist circumference by reducing 4 to 7 percent of your belly fat. It is ideal for people who want to lose weight, but want to preserve muscle mass, which is one way of improving your metabolism. Intermittent fasting can also improve insulin sensitivity, anti-aging, brain health, and reduce inflammation.

4. The Paleo Diet

Our ancestors live simply by gathering fresh food and cook them without processed ingredients contrary to what we are doing today. The simple food gathering and preparation by our hunter-gatherer forebears serves as an inspiration of the Paleo diet, which is believed to have extended the lives of our ancestors to hundred years. This popular diet program is based on the theory that the Western diet is linked to modern diseases and that our body is not intended to process grains, legumes, beans, meat and dairy as we are not machines.

Proponents of Paleo diet emphasized the consumption of whole foods (minimally processed), vegetables, fruits, lean meats (chicken, turkey), nuts and seeds. Consumption of processed and refined foods, including dairy, sugar, grains, are restricted, but other versions of Paleo diet limits the consumption of dairy products, such as milk and cheese. Some studies attest the positive effect of Paleo diet in reducing extra pounds and belly fat.

In a three-week study of 14 healthy individuals who followed a Paleo diet, it showed that there was an average of 5.1 pounds lost and their waist circumference had reduced by an average of 1.5 centimeters or 0.6 inches.

Another study revealed that this diet can offer satiation compared to other diet programs, such as low-fat diet and Mediterranean diet because of its high protein content, which can make your stomach, feel full. Its benefits to your health include reduction of risk for heart disease, such as cholesterol, triglyceride levels, and high blood pressure. Its downside is you are deprived of nutrients by restricting you to consume dairy, whole grains, legumes, and beans.

5. Low-Fat Diets

Followers of low-fat diets are restricted in their fat intake to thirty percent of their daily calories. Other versions of low-fat diets limit their followers to 10 percent below of calories from their fat consumption. Low-fat diets fat intake offers twice the amount of calories per gram compared to protein and carbohydrates. For followers of ultra-low-fat diets they are encourage to take fewer than ten percent calories from fat by getting 80 percent of calories from carbohydrates and ten percent from protein.

When we say ultra-low fat diets, they focus on eating a plant-based food sources and restrict meat and other meat products, such as eggs, dairy, and cheese. When it comes to weight loss, this diet can help a lot with its restrictions of calorie intake. A review of 33 studies involving 73,500 participants, it showed that there were significant changes in reducing weight and waist circumference.

Low-fat diets seem to be effective as low-carb diets in weight reduction in a controlled situation, but when it comes to everyday situations, the low-carb diets are more effective. Ultra-low-fat diets showed successful results in obese or overweight people. In fact, in an eight-week study involving 56 individuals, it showed that consumption of a diet composed of 7 to 14 percent fat resulted in an average weight reduction of 6.7 kilograms or 14.8 pounds.

The health benefits of taking low-fat diets include risk reduction of stroke and heart disease, alleviate inflammation and improve diabetes markers. The downside of restricting fat can also lead to some health issues in the future as fat helps in nutrient absorption, hormone production and cell development. A very-low-fat diet is linked to high risk of metabolic problems.

6. The DASH Diet

DASH stands for Dietary Approaches to Stop Hypertension, which is an eating plan geared at preventing and treating high blood pressure or hypertension. This diet puts emphasis on more consumption of fruits, vegetables, lean meats, and whole grains and should be low in salt, fat, added sugars and red meat. Although DASH diet is not strictly a weight loss diet, its followers claim, they were able to lose weight.

Dieters are encouraged to consume specific servings of a variety of food groups and the amount of servings depends on their recommended daily calorie intake. Under this program, you can eat about five servings of veggies, five servings of fruit, two servings of low-fat dairy products, two servings or fewer lean meats and seven servings of healthy carbohydrates from plant sources like whole grains each day. Nuts and seeds are allowed twice or thrice weekly. Studies show that the DASH diet is also effective in losing weight. A review of 13 studies shows that DASH dieters were able to lose more weight for more than 8 to 24 weeks compared to individuals who were put on a control diet. Its health benefits include reduction of risk factors of hypertension, colorectal and breast cancers. Since this diet emphasizes low salt, it can impact your health as it can also lead to increased insulin resistance and risk of death of individuals with heart disease.

7. The Mediterranean Diet

This diet is inspired by the diets of some people who live in Greece and Italy, which is believed to lower the risk of heart disease and aid in weight loss. Proponents of this diet emphasize the consumption of more vegetables, fruits, seeds, nuts, root crops, legumes, beans, fish, whole grains, seafood, and plant-based oils, such as extra-virgin olive or coconut oil. If you can't do away with poultry, dairy and eggs, you can eat them in moderation while red meat consumption is restricted.

Other foods that are restricted to a Mediterranean diet include trans fats, refined grains, processed meats, refined oils, added sugars and syrups, and other processed foods. Adopting this diet can help with weight loss as shown on a review of 19 studies, where participants were required to have a Mediterranean diet along with an exercise regimen or calorie restriction. The participants were able to lose an average of 4 kilograms or 8.8 pounds compared with those on a control diet.

The Mediterranean diet can fight infection, inflammation and oxidative stress. It also lowers the risk of cardiovascular disease and premature death due to stroke and heart attack. Since this diet is not totally a weight loss diet, you need to consume fewer calories to promote weight loss and better health.

8. WW Diet Program

WW was formerly called Weight Watchers, and one of the most followed weight loss programs as it does not restrict you from eating any of the food groups. If you adhere to this program, you are required to eat within your points set every day to reach your desired weight. Through its points-based system, this diet plan assigns a variety of foods and beverages a certain value based on their fiber, fat and calorie contents. You must stick to your daily point allowance to achieve your desired weight.

Numerous studies have revealed that this program can aid in weight loss. In a review of 45 studies, it revealed that individuals, who stick to their daily point allowance, were able to lose about 2.6 percent more weight compared to those people who had standard counseling. Individuals who stick to the programs were more successful in maintaining their weight for years than those who followed other diet programs. Since this diet allows flexibility, it can help those people with food intolerance and dietary restrictions. The downside of WW, is it can be expensive if you subscribe to a plan or some dieters would opt for unhealthy foods because it allows for flexibility.

Aside from the diets mentioned above, there are other diet programs that offer tons of health benefits and aid in weight loss. If you want to stay fit, choose a diet that is tailored to your food preferences, dietary restrictions and lifestyle to make sure you will stick to it. Before starting your diet plan, seek advice from your health care provider, especially if you are pregnant and have an existing illness.

Chapter 4: Foods to Help Build Lean Muscle

Most people are not aware that building a lean muscle is not only through physical activity, but it can also be achieved by eating certain foods. Your progress in muscle building depends on your intake of macronutrients, such as protein, carbohydrates and fats as your source of energy. If you desire to be in tip-top shape, focus on a regular strength training and bodyweight exercises and eat more calories every day.

Highly Recommended Foods to Build Muscles

1. Soybeans

Soybeans are great for increasing muscle growth and it is also a good source of iron, phosphorus and vitamin K. A half cup serving of cooked soybeans is packed with 14 grams of protein, vitamins, minerals, and healthy unsaturated fats.

2. Eggs

Eating eggs is best in gaining muscles as they are loaded with high-quality protein, vitamin B for energy production, choline, and healthy fats. The proteins in eggs are composed of large amounts of amino acid called leucine, which offer energy when exercising; help heals the skin and bones fast and help increase build lean body mass and muscle growth.

3. Turkey Breast

An alternative to chicken breast, turkey breast has high levels of vitamin B that can help increase muscle while supporting your body during exercise. It is also a good source of niacin, which aid in the processing of carbohydrates and fats in your body. A three-ounce serving of turkey breast is loaded with zero fat, zero carbohydrates and 25 grams of protein.

4. Salmon

Aside from its yummy taste, salmon is a great source of nutrients for muscle building, such as omega-3 fatty acids. A three-ounce serving of salmon is loaded with almost 2 grams of omega-3 fatty acids, 17 grams of protein and 5 grams of assortment of vitamin B.

5. Edamame

Immature beans called edamame are a great source of folate, protein, manganese and vitamin K. Folate functions in processing the amino acids in your body that can help increase muscle mass and strength. One cup of frozen edamame contains 8 grams of fiber for weight loss and 17 grams of protein for building lean muscle.

6. Chicken Breast

This favorite chicken part is high in protein for gaining muscle. Each three-ounce of serving is loaded with 26 grams of high-quality protein, and it also contains vitamin B6 and niacin, which are needed when you are physically active for optimal muscle growth and fat loss.

7. Greek Yogurt

Yogurt is a probiotic that contains a fast-digesting whey protein, high-quality protein and slow-digesting casein protein, which are essential in increasing lean muscle. Greek yogurt is highly recommended than ordinary yogurt because the amount of protein contents is double. If you are exercising, eat it after your workout or before sleeping.

8. Quinoa

When trying to build lean muscle, don't forget to include quinoa in your diet as your source of energy to get yourself active. Aside from carbohydrates, quinoa is high in magnesium, which plays a role in the normal functioning of your nerves and muscle. A cup of cooked quinoa contains 40 grams of carbohydrate, 5 grams of fiber, 8 grams of protein and high amounts of phosphorus and magnesium.

9. Tuna

Tuna takes pride of its large amounts of omega-3 fatty acids that aid in muscle health. Adults are advised to eat tuna as it helps slow down the loss of muscle mass and strength as they get older. A three-ounce serving of tuna has high amounts of all kinds of B vitamins, B12, B6, niacin and vitamin A for better exercise performance and energy.

10. Lean Beef

Consumption of lean beef can increase muscle mass while weight training because of its high quality protein, minerals, creatine, and vitamin B. Three ounces of 70 percent lean ground beef is loaded with

15 grams of fat and 228 calories. In another study, a three-ounce 95 percent lean ground beef is packed with more high quality protein with only 5 grams of fat and 145 calories.

11. Shrimp

Adding shrimp to your diet offers you muscle-building protein with fewer calories. It is loaded with amino acid leucine for muscle growth. A three-ounce serving of shrimp is loaded with 1 gram of fat, zero carbohydrates and 18 grams of protein.

12. Peanuts

Peanuts are high in amino acid leucine for building muscles compared to other plant foods. A half-cup serving of peanuts contain 425 calories, 16 grams carbohydrates, 17 grams protein, and large amounts of unsaturated fats.

13. Cottage Cheese

Cheese is a good source of muscle-building amino acid called leucine. Add this to your dish or snack food to meet your daily leucine requirements. A one cup serving of low-fat cottage cheese is packed with a high dose of leucine and 28 grams of protein.

14. Tilapia

If tuna is not available, substitute it with tilapia as your source of omega-3 fatty acids and vitamin B12 for your nerve and blood cell health, so that you can perform better in your body building exercise. A three-ounce serving offers high amounts of selenium, vitamin B12 and 21 grams of protein.

These are some foods that are recommended for building lean muscles and for losing weight. Most of these foods are packed with protein, leucine, omega-3 fatty acids, niacin, vitamin B12, and other nutrients to perform your exercise better and keep your body healthy. Just a reminder, focus on regular daily exercise and consume more calories every day from the above mentioned foods to reach your desired weight and lean muscle.

Conclusion

I hope this book "Healthy Eating to Gain Muscles & Healthy Weight" was able to help you learn about the importance of healthy eating, which involves mindful and slow eating to keep your body healthy. It also offers some popular diet programs and food varieties that can help build muscles and reduce weight.

The next step is to follow the contents of this book as your guide in weight loss and build muscle while doing some physical activities daily along with your chosen diet program, and incorporating the methodologies on how to begin mindful eating.

I hope you enjoyed reading this book as much as I enjoyed writing it!